The Mediterranean Diet for Beginners

Simple Mediterranean Recipes and 7 Day Meal Plan To Lose Weight, Increase Energy and Healthy Living

By

Anne Wilson

Table of Contents

Introduction

I want to thank you and congratulate you for purchasing the book, *"The Mediterranean Diet for Beginners: Simple Mediterranean Recipes and 7 Day Meal Plan To Lose Weight, Increase Energy and Healthy Living"*.

This book contains proven steps and strategies on how to start the Mediterranean diet.

If you want to live a long, healthy, and happy life, then it is high time for you to start following the Mediterranean Diet. Why? This healthy diet is scientifically proven to reduce your risk of developing heart disease, certain types of cancer, and type 2 diabetes.

Let this book help you out on how to get started on the Mediterranean diet in the most healthy and affordable way possible!

Thanks again for purchasing this book, I hope you enjoy it!

CHAPTER 1

Beginner's Guide to the Mediterranean Diet

Although most people nowadays call it the Mediterranean diet, it is actually considered as the ideal lifestyle by the people in the Mediterranean countries. It is even touted as the healthiest diet in the world for four main reasons.

First, those who follow the Mediterranean diet regard food as medicine. Any ingredient that is not natural is generally avoided, and even whole foods that are scientifically proven to cause adverse effects on the body if consumed regularly are avoided or eaten only in small portions.

Second is that it is not just about what you eat, but also about how active you should be. In other words, engaging in regular physical activities is a must in the Mediterranean lifestyle.

It is important to keep your body moving for it to stay healthy, such as by gardening, swimming, going out for regular walks, and so on. When you spend time with other people, you get to enjoy life more. Bond with the family by preparing meals together; this will make cooking more fun and less laborious.

Set aside a special time of the day to exercise. Let it be a time not just to help strengthen and tone your body but also a moment when you can reflect. You might also enjoy the occasional company of friends during your workout sessions.

Third is that social lifestyle is highlighted. In the Mediterranean diet, it is considered to be unhealthy to eat alone. When you really stop to think about it, you get to savor your food more and eat more slowly when you are interacting with a meal buddy.

The last reason is that the diet emphasizes the concept of moderation. An ingredient, no matter how healthy it is, should still be eaten in moderation. Wine and olive oil, which are staple parts of the diet, should also be consumed in moderation.

All of these principles in the Mediterranean diet are what make it a healthy one. When you keep these in mind constantly, you will notice that you will be more mindful of your food choices and your meal times will become more enjoyable.

The Food Pyramid of the Mediterranean Diet

There are five tiers in the food pyramid of the Mediterranean Diet. It is important to remember this food pyramid as it will be your guide in choosing what to put on your plate. Here it is:

Tier 1: Regular Social and Physical Activities

That's right, the biggest tier in the pyramid is dedicated not to food but to relationships with others and with yourself.

Tier 2: Vegetables, Fruit, Whole Grains, Beans, Legumes, Seeds, Nuts, Herbs, Spices, and Olive oil

The bulk on your plate should consist mostly of vegetables with the rest sprinkled on top. In layman's terms, go green with a rainbow of colors on top. This is a stark contrast to the typical Western diet, which consists mostly of red meat and starchy sides.

Tier 3: Fish and Seafood

If you feel the need to eat meat, then always choose seafood first, especially wild-caught fish. In the diet, fish should be served at least twice a week.

Tier 4: Eggs, Yogurt, Cheese, and Poultry

Eggs and dairy products can be enjoyed regularly in the Mediterranean diet, but it is emphasized that they should only be served in small portions.

Tier 5: Meat and Sweets

People in the Mediterranean diet are not in the habit of slaughtering their farm animals unless it is a special occasion, so meats do not play a central role in their diet. If they do serve meat, they make sure to have plenty of vegetables with it. Sweets are also enjoyed on special occasions, such as once a week.

At first, it might seem difficult to constantly have to buy fresh whole foods, but when you plan ahead, everything will be so much easier. It also would not hurt to grow some of your own. Many people have learned to grow herbs and spices, for instance. When you want to eat these healthy ingredients for the rest of your life, a little goes a long way!

CHAPTER 2

The 7-Day Meal Plan

You can think of this 7-day meal plan as more of a suggestion than a set of rules, especially if you decide to cook for one. This meal plan is ideal for those who would like to spend more time in the kitchen and are cooking for two or more.

However, if you are cooking for one, then the recommendation would be for you to choose a favorite set, prepare the dishes in bulk, and pack them up in the kitchen so that all you will have to do is reheat and enjoy throughout the week. Of course, if you still wish to prepare your own meals each day, then all the better. The Mediterranean diet is all about eating a variety of healthy and delicious food made up of fresh ingredients. After all, your health and happiness are all worth the extra effort.

Day 1
Breakfast: Italian Basil and Mushroom Omelet
Lunch: Provençal Vegetable Soup
Dinner: Steamed Italian Halibut with Green Grapes
Side Dish: Tender Roasted Sweet Potatoes with Savory Tahini Sauce

Day 2
Breakfast: Mediterranean Fruit Oatmeal
Lunch: Grilled Chicken Salad with Fennel, Orange, and Raisins
Dinner: Hearty Root Veggie and Beef Stew
Side Dish: Homemade Whole Wheat Pita Bread

Day 3
Breakfast: Smoked Salmon and Asparagus Omelet
Lunch: Simple Rosemary Shrimp Polenta
Dinner: Italian Chicken Stew with Potatoes, Bell Peppers and Tomatoes
Side Dish: Crisp Spiced Cauliflower with Feta Cheese

Day 4
Breakfast: Mediterranean Muesli
Lunch: Tunisian Turnovers with Tuna, Egg and Tomato
Dinner: Eggplants with Tomato and Minced Lamb Stuffing
Side Dish: Pumpkin Kibbeh

Day 5
Breakfast: Buckwheat Berry Crepes with Cottage Cheese
Lunch: Fish and Spinach Gratin
Dinner: Savory Roasted Sea Bass
Side Dish: Oven Roasted Carrots with Olives and Cumin Yogurt Sauce

Day 6
Breakfast: No-Crust Broccoli and Cheese Quiche
Lunch: Calamari with Herb and Rice Stuffing
Dinner: Pork Roast with Zest Fig and Acorn Squash
Side Dish: Bravas Potatoes with Roasted Tomato Sauce

Day 7
Breakfast: Banana-Strawberry Breakfast Smoothie
Lunch: Classic Niçoise Chicken
Dinner: Warm-Spiced Lamb Meatballs in Tomato Sauce
Side Dish: Spring Peas and Beans with Zesty Thyme Yogurt Sauce

CHAPTER 3

Breakfast Recipes

Italian Basil and Mushroom Omelet

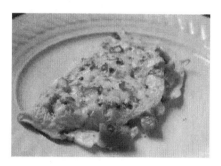

Makes: 2 servings

Ingredients:

- ❖ 2 Tbsp. extra virgin olive oil
- ❖ 1/2 small yellow onion, sliced thinly into rounds
- ❖ 3 large eggs
- ❖ 1 small leek, white and light green parts, chopped
- ❖ 1 cup shiitake mushrooms, stemmed and sliced thinly
- ❖ 4 fresh basil leaves
- ❖ 1/2 tsp. sea salt
- ❖ 2 Tbsp. grated Pecorino Romano cheese

Instructions:

1. Whisk the eggs in a bowl until foamy, then set aside.

2. Place a skillet over medium high flame and heat the olive oil. Sauté the onion until tender.

3. Stir in the mushrooms and sauté until browned. Stir in the leeks and sauté until tender.

4. Stir in the basil leaves, then pour in half the beaten egg. Reduce to medium low flame, cover the skillet and cook until the eggs are almost set.

5. With a spatula, gently lift the omelet and pour in the remaining egg beneath. Sprinkle the cheese and salt on top, then cover again and cook for 3 minutes, or until set.

6. Transfer the omelet on a platter, slice in half, then serve right away.

Smoked Salmon and Asparagus Omelet

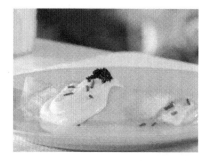

Makes: 2 servings

Ingredients:

- ❖ 1 tsp. canola oil

- ❖ 1/2 Tbsp. minced onion

- ❖ 1/2 tsp. minced garlic

- ❖ 4 steamed asparagus spears

- ❖ 2 sliced smoked salmon, chopped

- ❖ 4 eggs

- ❖ 1/2 tsp. freshly squeezed lemon juice

- ❖ 1 Tbsp. minced fresh flat leaf parsley

- ❖ 1/2 tsp. minced fresh dill

- ❖ 1/2 tsp. minced fresh chives

- ❖ 1/2 Tbsp. milk

- ❖ Sea salt

- ❖ Freshly ground black pepper

Instructions:

1. Place a skillet over medium flame and heat the canola oil.

2. Sauté the onion until tender, then stir in the asparagus and garlic. Sauté until fragrant, then add the lemon juice and mix well. Spread the asparagus spears in an even layer on the skillet.

3. Whisk together the milk, eggs, parsley, dill, and chives. Season with salt and pepper, then pour into the skillet.

4. Sprinkle the chopped smoked salmon all over the mixture, then cover the skillet and reduce flame to low. Cook for 2 minutes, or until eggs are set.

5. Carefully flip over with a spatula and cook for 1 minute. Transfer to a plate, slice in half, then serve right away.

No-Crust Broccoli and Cheese Quiche

Makes: 4 servings

Ingredients:

- ❖ 1 tsp. extra virgin olive oil
- ❖ 3 large eggs
- ❖ 3 scallions, sliced
- ❖ 1 cup chopped broccoli florets
- ❖ 1/4 cup light cream

- ❖ 1/3 tsp. dried tarragon
- ❖ 1/4 cup mild goat cheese
- ❖ 1/4 cup grated Gruyere
- ❖ Sea salt
- ❖ Freshly ground black pepper

Instructions:

1. Set the oven to 350 degrees F. Lightly oil a mini pie plate with olive oil.

2. Heat the remaining olive oil in a skillet over medium flame. Stir in the scallions and sauté until tender. Stir in the broccoli and sauté until tender, about 6 minutes. Turn off the heat and set aside to cool slightly.

3. Beat the eggs, tarragon, and light cream in a bowl, then season with salt and pepper. Add the cheeses and broccoli, mixing well.

4. Pour the mixture into the prepared pie plate and bake for 25 to 30 minutes, or until firm and golden. Serve warm.

Mediterranean Fruit Oatmeal

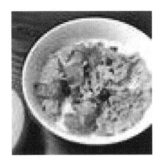

Makes: 2 servings

Ingredients:

* ❖ 1 cup old fashioned oats

* ❖ 1/2 apple, cored, peeled and minced

* ❖ 1/2 mango, peeled and diced

* ❖ 2 cups hot milk

* ❖ 2 tsp. chopped almonds

* ❖ 2 tsp. sunflower seeds

Instructions:

1. Combine the oats and hot milk in a bowl. Cover and set aside for 2 minutes.

2. Fold the chopped almonds and sunflower seeds into the mixture,

3. Fold in the mango and apple, then serve right away.

Mediterranean Muesli

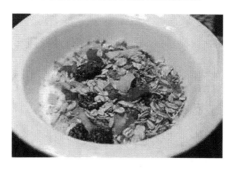

Makes: 2 servings

Ingredients:

* ❖ 2 Tbsp. raisins

* ❖ 2 Tbsp. dried berries

* ❖ 2 tsp. chopped walnuts

* ❖ 2 tsp. chopped almonds

* ❖ 1 cup muesli cereal

* ❖ 1 cup Greek yogurt

Instructions:

1. Combine the muesli cereal and yogurt in a bowl.

2. Fold in the almonds, walnuts, raisins, and berries, then serve right away.

Buckwheat Berry Crepes with Cottage Cheese

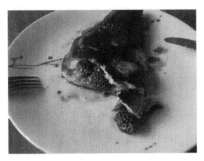

Makes: 3 to 4 servings

Ingredients:

- ❖ 1/4 cup buckwheat flour
- ❖ 1/4 cup all-purpose flour
- ❖ 1 egg
- ❖ 1 Tbsp. grape-seed oil
- ❖ 1/2 Tbsp. maple syrup
- ❖ 1 Tbsp. melted unsalted butter
- ❖ 1/2 cup milk
- ❖ 4 oz low fat cottage cheese
- ❖ 1/2 tsp. vanilla extract
- ❖ 1 cup fresh berries
- ❖ Sea salt
- ❖ Maple syrup for serving

Instructions:

1. In a mixing bowl, combine the buckwheat flour and all purpose flour. Set aside.

2. In a small bowl, whisk the egg until foamy, then whisk in the grape-seed oil, maple syrup, vanilla extract, and a small pinch of salt. Gradually mix in the milk.

3. Cove r the bowl with a clean kitchen towel and set aside for half an hour.

4. To cook the crepes, place a crepe pan or non-stick griddle over medium flame and heat through. Lightly oil the pan with a bit of grape-seed oil.

5. Add a bit of water to the batter if it is too thick; the consistency should be smooth and a bit runny.

6. Spoon the batter on the hot pan and swirl to spread. Cook for 1 minute or until firm, then carefully flip over with a crepe spatula. Cook until golden, then place on a platter.

7. Once all the crepes are cooked, spread the cottage cheese evenly over each crepe, then sprinkle the berries evenly over each. Roll up and arrange on a plate.

8. Drizzle maple syrup on top, then serve right away.

Banana-Strawberry Breakfast Smoothie

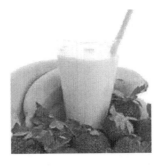

Makes: 3 servings

Ingredients:

- ❖ 2 cups crushed ice
- ❖ 2 ripe bananas
- ❖ 1 1/2 cups sliced strawberries
- ❖ 1 1/2 cups Greek yogurt
- ❖ 3 Tbsp. flaxseeds
- ❖ 3 Tbsp. organic honey

Instructions:

1. Blend the ice, yogurt, honey, and banana in a blender on high speed until smooth.

2. Add the flaxseeds and strawberries and blend on low speed until smooth.

3. Pour the smoothie into three glasses and serve right away.

CHAPTER 4

Lunch Recipes

Provençal Vegetable Soup

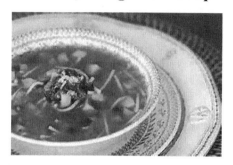

Makes: 3 servings

Ingredients:

❖ 1/2 Tbsp. olive oil

❖ 1 small onion, chopped

❖ 1/2 cup chopped green beans

❖ 1/2 cup dry red beans

❖ 1/2 cup dry white beans

❖ 1 carrot, chopped

❖ 1 small zucchini, chopped

❖ 1/2 medium leek, trimmed and chopped

❖ 2 medium tomatoes

❖ 1 large potato, peeled and chopped

❖ 3 garlic cloves, minced

❖ 1 sage leaf

❖ 2 Tbsp. chopped fresh flat leaf parsley

❖ 1/2 cup whole wheat penne pasta

❖ Sea salt

❖ Freshly ground black pepper

For the Pesto:

❖ 3 garlic cloves

❖ 1/2 cup fresh basil, packed

❖ 2 Tbsp. olive oil

❖ 1/4 cup shredded Parmesan cheese

Instructions:

1. Pour the red and white beans in a pot, then pour enough water to cover them by about an inch.

2. Place the pot over high flame, cover, and bring to a boil. Once boiling. Turn off the heat and set aside for an hour.

3. Prepare the pesto by combining the garlic, basil, cheese, and 1/2 tablespoon olive oil in the food processor. Pulse until pasty, then drizzle in the olive oil and blend until smooth. Refrigerate until ready to serve.

4. Ensure that the vegetables are all chopped in the same size.

5. Prepare the penne pasta based on the manufacturer's directions, then drain and toss in a bit of olive oil. Set aside.

6. Boil salted water in a small saucepan and blanch the tomatoes until tender. Immediately drain and plunge in a bowl of ice water. Skin the tomatoes, then remove the seeds and chop up. Set aside.

7. Place a soup pot over high flame and heat the olive oil. Sauté the onions until tender, then stir in the garlic, chopped tomatoes, and leek. Sauté until simmering and garlic is fragrant.

8. Add the red and white beans, green beans, zucchini, carrot, potato, parsley, and sage, then add just enough water to cover them. Bring to a boil, then reduce to low flame.

9. Cover the pot and simmer for 30 minutes, or until the vegetables are fork tender. If desired, puree the potatoes and mix into the soup.

10. Mix in the pasta, then season to taste with salt and pepper. Serve the soup with the pesto on the side.

Simple Rosemary Shrimp Polenta

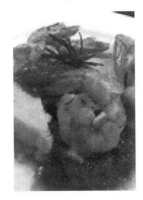

Makes: 3 servings

Ingredients:

- ❖ 2 Tbsp. extra virgin olive oil

- ❖ 1 1/2 cups cooked polenta

- ❖ 1 tsp. chopped fresh rosemary

- ❖ 3/4 cup large shrimp, peeled and deveined

- ❖ 1 garlic clove, minced

- ❖ 1/4 tsp. sea salt

- ❖ 1/8 tsp. freshly ground black pepper

- ❖ Crushed red chili flakes

Instructions:

1. Place a skillet over medium high flame and heat the olive oil.

2. Sauté the garlic until fragrant, then stir in the shrimp, salt, pepper, rosemary, and a dash of red chili flakes. Sauté until shrimp is pink and cooked through.

3. Spread the polenta on a serving bowl, packing down gently. Spoon the rosemary shrimp on top, then serve right away.

Grilled Chicken Salad with Fennel, Orange, and Raisins

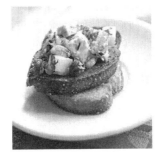

Makes: 3 servings

Ingredients:

- ❖ 1/4 cup extra virgin olive oil

- ❖ 1 tsp. Dijon mustard

- ❖ 1/2 lb. boneless, skinless chicken breast

- ❖ 1 Tbsp. freshly squeezed lemon juice

- ❖ 1/4 cup freshly squeezed orange juice

- ❖ 1 small fennel bulb, trimmed and chopped

- ❖ 1 Tbsp. minced fresh mint

- ❖ 1 tsp. Dijon mustard

- ❖ 1 1/2 Tbsp. golden raisins

- ❖ 2 1/2 Tbsp. warm water

- ❖ 1 Boston Bibb lettuce, rinsed and spun dry

- ❖ 1 small orange, peeled and divided into segments

❖ Sea salt

❖ Freshly ground black pepper

For the vinaigrette:

❖ 1 Tbsp. balsamic vinegar

❖ 3 Tbsp. extra virgin olive oil

Instructions:

1. Blend the orange juice, lemon juice, mint, olive oil, and mustard in a bowl. Season to taste with salt and pepper.

2. Add the chicken breast in the mixture and turn several times to coat. Cover the bowl and refrigerate for at least an hour.

3. Take the bowl out of the refrigerator and set aside for 15 minutes.

4. Prepare the grill.

5. Soak the raisins in the warm water until plump.

6. Grill the chicken over medium high flame until cooked through, about 6 to 8 minutes per side depending on the thickness.

7. While the chicken is grilling, grill the fennel for about 6 minutes and the orange segments for about 3 minutes or until tender. Baste the chicken, fennel, and orange with the marinade all the time.

8. Transfer the grilled ingredients to a platter and set aside.

9. Place the lettuce and mint on a serving dish. Drain the raisins and set aside.

10. Prepare the vinaigrette by blending the balsamic vinegar and olive oil. Season with salt and pepper to taste.

11. Chop up the grilled chicken breast, fennel, and orange. Arrange on top of the lettuce, then scatter the raisins and drizzle the dressing on top. Serve right away.

Tunisian Turnovers with Tuna, Egg and Tomato

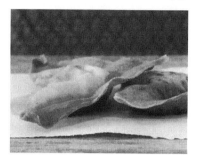

Makes: 2 servings

Ingredients:

❖ 2 pieces pita bread (See Chapter 6: *Homemade Whole Wheat Pita Bread*)

❖ 2 Tbsp. extra virgin olive oil

❖ 5 oz. tuna packed in olive oil, drained

❖ 1 hard-boiled egg, sliced thinly

❖ 1 large ripe tomato, sliced thinly

❖ 1 small ripe tomato, diced

❖ 1 garlic clove, minced

❖ 1/4 small green bell pepper, seeded and minced

❖ 1/4 small yellow onion, minced

❖ 1/2 small English cucumber, sliced extra thin

❖ 1/4 cup pitted black olives

❖ 2 Tbsp. hot sauce

❖ 2 jarred pepperoncini peppers, drained and halved

❖ Sea salt

❖ Freshly ground black pepper

Instructions:

1. Place a skillet over medium high flame and heat the olive oil. Saute the onion, tomato, garlic, and bell pepper until tender and simmering. Season to taste with salt and pepper, then turn off the heat.

2. Open up the pita bread and spoon the tomato sauce inside, then add cucumber slices, tuna, olives, pepperoncini pepper, and egg.

3. Arrange on a platter and server right away with hot sauce on the side.

Classic Niçoise Chicken

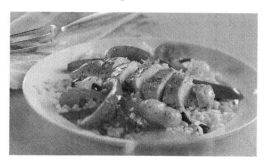

Makes: 4 servings

Ingredients:

- ❖ 2 lb chicken breasts or legs, excess skin and fat removed
- ❖ 3 Tbsp. extra virgin olive oil
- ❖ 2 small onions, chopped
- ❖ 1 garlic clove, minced
- ❖ 1/2 Tbsp. minced fresh thyme
- ❖ 3 ripe tomatoes, chopped
- ❖ 1/4 cup small black olives
- ❖ 1/4 cup vermouth or dry white wine
- ❖ 1/4 cup chopped fresh flat leaf parsley
- ❖ 2 Tbsp. freshly squeezed lemon juice
- ❖ Sea salt
- ❖ Freshly ground black pepper

Instructions:

1. Season the chicken pieces all over with salt and pepper, then set aside.

2. Heat 1 1/2 tablespoons of oil in a heavy bottomed skillet over medium flame. Brown the chicken all over, approximately 6 minutes per side.

3. Meanwhile, place another skillet over medium flame and heat 1 1/2 tablespoons of olive oil.

4. Sauté the onion until tender, then stir in the garlic and sauté until golden. Stir in the parsley and thyme and sauté until fragrant. Turn off the heat and set aside.

5. Stir the tomatoes and vermouth or wine into the chicken pieces, scraping up the bottom to loosen any browned bits.

6. Set the flame to medium high, then simmer, uncovered, for about 15 to 20 minutes or until the sauce is thickened. The chicken must be cooked through.

7. Add the herb mixture in with the chicken, then mix well. Add the olives and lemon juice, then let everything boil for about 3 minutes.

8. Transfer the dish to a plate and serve right away.

Calamari with Herb and Rice Stuffing

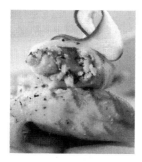

Makes: 6 servings

Ingredients:

- ❖ 3 Tbsp. extra virgin olive oil
- ❖ 3 cups vegetable or seafood broth
- ❖ 1/3 cup uncooked short grain rice
- ❖ 1 1/2 small yellow onions, minced
- ❖ 1 1/2 lb. fresh spinach
- ❖ 3 Tbsp. chopped fresh flat leaf parsley
- ❖ 3 Tbsp. chopped fresh dill
- ❖ 1 1/2 lb. baby squid
- ❖ 1 1/2 tsp. sea salt
- ❖ Freshly ground black pepper
- ❖ Red chili flakes

Instructions:

1. Place a large skillet over medium flame and heat 1 1/2 tablespoons of olive oil. Stir in the onion and sauté until tender and golden brown.

2. Stir in the parsley, dill, rice, and spinach, then season with salt, pepper, and red chili flakes. Simmer for about a minute, then turn off the heat. Let the mixture cool down slightly.

3. Remove the tentacles from the baby squid, then rinse the squid well. Stuff each squid with the rice mixture, then secure the ends with the toothpick. Ensure that there is space inside the squid for the rice to puff up later on.

4. Heat the rest of the olive oil in a skillet over medium flame, then add the calamari and cook until browned all over.

5. Pour the broth into the skillet, then cover and reduce to low flame. Simmer for up to 20 minutes, or until the rice inside the calamari is completely puffed and tender. Best served warm.

Fish and Spinach Gratin

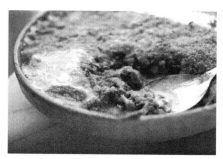

Makes: 3 servings

Ingredients:

- ❖ 1 Tbsp. extra virgin olive oil

- ❖ 3/4 lb firm white fish fillets

- ❖ 1 lb fresh spinach, rinsed thoroughly

- ❖ 1 small onion, chopped

- ❖ 1/2 Tbsp. Dijon mustard

- ❖ 1 small garlic clove, chopped

- ❖ 2 Tbsp. freshly squeezed lemon juice

- ❖ 1/3 cup ground dry unseasoned bread crumbs

- ❖ Sea salt

- ❖ Freshly ground black pepper

Instructions:

1. Rinse the spinach thoroughly under cold running water.

2. Place a dry saucepan over medium flame and add the spinach. Cover and cook the spinach for about 8 minutes or until wilted. Remove from heat, chop, and set aside.

3. Wipe the saucepan clean and place it over medium low flame. Heat 1/2 tablespoon of olive oil and sauté the onion until tender. Add the garlic and sauté until fragrant.

4. Add the Dijon mustard and wilted spinach and sauté until thoroughly combined. Season with salt and pepper to taste. Turn off the heat and set aside.

5. Set the oven to 450 degrees F. Coat a small casserole or gratin dish with the remaining olive oil.

6. Wash the fish fillets thoroughly, then blot dry with paper towels and season both sides with salt and pepper.

7. Spread half of the spinach mixture on the dish in an even layer, then place the fish fillets on top. Sprinkle the lemon juice all over.

8. Add the remaining spinach mixture in an even layer on top, then sprinkle the bread crumbs all over.

9. Bake for 15 to 20 minutes, or until the fish is cooked through. Serve right away.

CHAPTER 5

Dinner Recipes

Steamed Italian Halibut with Green Grapes

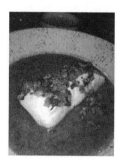

Makes: 2 servings

Ingredients:

- ❖ 2 boneless halibut fillets, approximately 4 oz each

- ❖ 2 Tbsp. extra virgin olive oil

- ❖ 1 cup seedless green grapes

- ❖ 2 garlic cloves, chopped

- ❖ 1/2 small red chili pepper, minced

- ❖ 1/4 tsp. sea salt

- ❖ Freshly ground black pepper

- ❖ 1/4 cup torn fresh basil leaves

- ❖ 3/4 cup water

Instructions:

1. Place a large, deep, heavy duty skillet over medium high flame and heat the olive oil.

2. Add the halibut fillets in a single layer, then scatter the garlic, chili pepper, basil, and grapes around them. Season with salt and pepper.

3. Pour the water around the fillets, then cover the skillet and reduce to medium low flame.

4. Simmer for 7 minutes, then uncover and flip the fillets over. Cover again and simmer for an additional 5 to 7 minutes, or until the fillets are cooked through.

5. Carefully transfer the fish onto a platter and cover to keep warm.

6. Increase the heat under the skillet to medium high, then simmer the liquids until saucy and flavorful. Adjust seasonings to taste, then spoon the mixture over the fillets and serve right away.

Italian Chicken Stew with Potatoes, Bell Peppers and Tomatoes

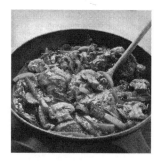

Makes: 6 servings

Ingredients:

- ❖ 1/3 cup extra virgin olive oil

- ❖ 3 Yukon gold potatoes, peeled and sliced into thin rounds

- ❖ 3 garlic cloves, minced

- ❖ 2 medium onions, chopped

- ❖ 2 medium red bell peppers, seeded and chopped

- ❖ 2 medium green bell peppers, seeded and chopped

- ❖ 3 cups diced tomatoes

- ❖ 3 Tbsp. chopped fresh basil

- ❖ 3 Tbsp. chopped fresh flat leaf parsley

- ❖ 1/3 tsp. crushed red pepper

- ❖ 1/3 tsp. freshly ground black pepper

- ❖ 1 1/2 lb boneless chicken breast, cubed

Instructions:

1. Place a heavy duty stew pot over medium flame and heat 4 1/2 tablespoons of olive oil. Stir in the cubed chicken and saute until browned all over. Transfer to a plate lined with paper towels using a slotted spoon.

2. Heat the rest of the olive oil in the stew pot, then stir in the onion and bell peppers. Saute until tender, then add the garlic. Saute until garlic is fragrant.

3. Return the browned chicken into the pot and stir in the salt, pepper, crushed red pepper, basil, parsley, and tomatoes. Mix well.

4. Set high flame and bring mixture to a boil. Once boiling, reduce to medium low and mix well. Cover and simmer for up to 25 minutes.

5. Uncover and mix in the potatoes, then cover again and simmer for about 45 minutes or until potatoes are tender. Serve warm.

Eggplants with Tomato and Minced Lamb Stuffing

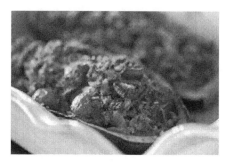

Makes: 3 servings

Ingredients:

- ❖ 3/4 lb finely minced shoulder of lamb

- ❖ 3 small eggplants, sliced in half

- ❖ 1 onion, minced

- ❖ 2 garlic cloves

- ❖ 1/2 tsp. freshly ground toasted black peppercorns

- ❖ 1/2 tsp. ground cinnamon

- ❖ 1/2 tsp. ground cardamom pods

- ❖ 1/2 tsp. ground whole cloves

- ❖ 1/2 tsp. chili flakes

- ❖ 1 1/2 cups San Marzano tomatoes, crushed

- ❖ 1/4 cup toasted pine nuts

- ❖ 1 tsp. muscovado sugar

❖ 2 Tbsp. chopped fresh flat leaf parsley

❖ Olive oil

❖ Sea salt

Instructions:

1. Set the oven to 425 degrees F.

2. Place the eggplant halves on a baking dish with the exposed side facing upward. Coat the eggplants with a bit of olive oil, then sprinkle salt on top.

3. Bake the eggplants for 15 minutes, or until tender.

4. Carefully take the eggplants out of the oven and cut pockets in their center to place the stuffing in; be careful not to cut all the way through. Cover and set aside.

5. Using a mortar and pestle or food processor, crush the garlic into a paste. Set aside.

6. Place a skillet over medium flame and heat about half a tablespoon of olive oil. Saute the onion until tender, then stir in the garlic paste and saute until fragrant.

7. Stir the minced lamb into the skillet, then add the spices and saute until lamb is browned and cooked through.

8. Fold the pine nuts and crushed tomatoes into the meat mixture, then stir in the muscovado sugar and a pinch of salt.

9. Set oven temperature to 350 degrees F. Line the baking dish with aluminum foil and set aside.

10. Stuff the eggplants with the meat and tomato mixture. Arrange on the prepared baking dish, then bake for about 25 to 30 minutes, or until eggplant is completely tender.

11. Place the eggplants on a platter, top with parsley, and serve right away.

Pork Roast with Zest Fig and Acorn Squash

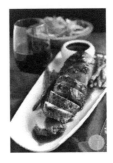

Makes: 6 servings

Ingredients:

- ❖ 30 oz boneless pork loin roast
- ❖ 1 1/2 cups chicken or vegetable stock
- ❖ 4 1/2 Tbsp. minced fresh flat leaf parsley
- ❖ 2 fresh rosemary sprigs
- ❖ 1 1/2 tsp. olive oil
- ❖ 3 Tbsp. chopped almonds
- ❖ Sea salt
- ❖ Freshly ground black pepper

For the Figs

- ❖ 12 figs
- ❖ 2 cups freshly squeezed orange or lemon juice
- ❖ 3 acorn squash

- ❖ 2/3 cup Chardonnay
- ❖ 3 Tbsp. honey

Instructions:

1. Set the oven 350 degrees F.

2. Score the figs, then place on a baking dish. Halve the acorn squash and remove the seeds, then arrange next to the figs. Set aside.

3. Pour the orange or lemon juice into a saucepan, then place over high flame and stir in the Chardonnay and honey. Bring to a boil.

4. Once boiling, pour the mixture over the acorn squash and figs. Bake for half an hour.

5. To roast the pig, first prepare the broiler.

6. Place the pork roast on a roasting pan, then massage the olive oil all over it. Season with salt and pepper, then broil for about an hour or until the internal temperature of the roast is at least 185 degrees F.

7. Transfer the roast to a platter and cover to keep warm.

8. Pour the stock into the roasting pan and scrape to loosen up the browned bits of roast on the pan. Pour the mixture into a saucepan.

9. Place the saucepan with the stock and browned bits over high flame and bring to a boil. Once boiling, reduce to a simmer, then stir in the rosemary. Continue to simmer as you pour the liquids from the baked figs and acorn squash. Simmer until thickened.

10. Carve the pork roast, then spoon the roasted figs and acorn squash on the side. Drizzle the sauce all over, then add the almonds and serve right away.

Savory Roasted Sea Bass

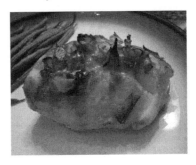

Makes: 6 servings

Ingredients:

- ❖ 3 whole sea bass (or snapper), 2 lb each

- ❖ 1 whole garlic bulb, peeled

- ❖ 3 sun-dried tomatoes

- ❖ 3 cups fresh flat leaf parsley

- ❖ 3 cups fresh cilantro

- ❖ 4 1/2 Tbsp. toasted cumin seeds

- ❖ 1 1/2 Tbsp. sweet smoked paprika

- ❖ 1/3 cup freshly squeezed lemon juice

- ❖ 2 1/2 tsp. ground chilies

- ❖ 2 small lemons

- ❖ 2/3 cup extra virgin olive oil

- ❖ Sea salt

Instructions:

1. Have the fish cleaned and gutted at the fishmonger's if you cannot do it yourself.

2. Blend together the parsley, garlic, cilantro, sun-dried tomatoes, paprika, lemon juice, cumin, and chilies in a food processor. Season to taste with salt, then drizzle in just enough olive oil as you pulse until the mixture becomes pasty.

3. Set the oven to 425 degrees F. Cover a rimmed baking sheet with baking paper and set aside.

4. Trim off the fins of the fish, then form 2 inch deep pockets in both sides of each fish. Drizzle the remaining olive oil all over the fish and rub gently to coat, including the insides of the pockets.

5. Spoon the herb and spice paste into the pockets of the fish, then arrange the fish on the prepared baking sheet.

6. Roast for half an hour, or until the fish are cooked through.

7. Transfer the roasted fish to a platter, then slice the lemons in half and squeezed the juices over the fish just before serving.

Warm-Spiced Lamb Meatballs in Tomato Sauce

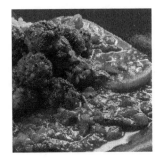

Makes: 3 servings

Ingredients:

- ❖ 3 garlic cloves, chopped

- ❖ 1 small yellow onion, quartered

- ❖ 1 lb finely minced lamb

- ❖ 1/2 tsp. cinnamon

- ❖ 1/2 tsp. ground cumin

- ❖ 1/4 tsp. sea salt

- ❖ 1/8 tsp. freshly ground black pepper

For the Tomato Sauce:

- ❖ 1/2 Tbsp. pure olive oil

- ❖ 2 cups pureed tomato

- ❖ 1/2 small onion, minced

- ❖ 2 garlic cloves, minced

- ❖ 1/2 cinnamon stick

- ❖ Sea salt

- ❖ Freshly ground black pepper

Instructions:

1. Prepare the broiler.

2. In a food processor, process the minced lamb with the cumin, cinnamon, salt, pepper, onion, and garlic until pasty.

3. Transfer the meat mixture onto a clean, dry work surface, then divide into 6 large meatballs. Roll out until about 2 1/2 inches in length and an inch in width.

4. Arrange the meatballs on a baking sheet, then broil for 3 minutes per side, or until golden brown and cooked through. Remove from the broiler and set aside.

5. Make the sauce by placing a saucepan over medium flame. Heat the olive oil and saute the onion until golden. Add the garlic and saute until fragrant.

6. Stir the pureed tomato into the pan, then add the cinnamon stick, salt, and pepper. Increase heat until mixture boils, then reduce to low flame.

7. Place the meatballs into the sauce and mix well. Cover the pan, then simmer for about 12 minutes or until the sauce thickens. Best served warm.

Hearty Root Veggie and Beef Stew

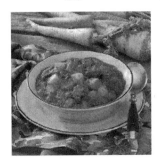

Makes: 3 servings

Ingredients:

- ❖ 2 lb beef short ribs, excess fat removed
- ❖ 6 small potatoes, scrubbed
- ❖ 1 carrot, peeled and chopped
- ❖ 1 parsnip, peeled and chopped
- ❖ 3 turnips, peeled and halved
- ❖ 4 cups chicken broth or water
- ❖ 1 yellow onion, chopped
- ❖ 1/4 cup chopped garlic
- ❖ 2 Tbsp. freshly grated ginger
- ❖ 1 tsp. ground ginger
- ❖ 1/2 cinnamon stick
- ❖ 1/2 Tbsp. freshly ground toasted black peppercorns

- ❖ 1/2 Tbsp. smoked sweet paprika

- ❖ 2 star anise

- ❖ 1 bay leaf

- ❖ 1/2 Tbsp. freshly squeezed lemon juice

- ❖ 2 Tbsp. chopped fresh cilantro

- ❖ Sea salt

- ❖ Canola oil

Instructions:

1. Set the oven to 325 degrees F.

2. Sprinkle salt all over the beef and set aside.

3. Place an oven-proof pot over medium flame and heat just enough canola oil to cover the bottom.

4. Increase to medium high flame and cook the beef until browned all over. Place the browned beef on a baking sheet and set aside.

5. In the same pot, stir in the onion, ginger, and garlic over medium flame. Saute until onion is tender, then stir in the ginger powder, spices, and black peppercorns for about a minute.

6. Pour a bit of the broth or water into the pot, then scrape the bottom to loosen up any browned bits.

7. Place the bay leaf and cilantro into a tea bag and add into the pot. Add the beef back into the pot, then pour in the remaining broth or water.

8. Increase to a boil, then cover and transfer to the oven. Cook for 1 hour, or until the beef is extra tender.

9. While the soup is in the oven, toss together all of the chopped root vegetables in a bowl with some salt and oil. Spread the vegetables on a baking sheet lined with baking paper, then roast in the oven for half an hour, or until almost tender.

10. At the end of 1 hour, remove the pot from the oven and take the beef out. Place on a platter and keep covered.

11. Set the soup aside for 8 minutes, then remove the solidified fat on the surface. Discard the tea bag of herbs, star anise, and cinnamon stick.

12. Stir the roasted vegetables into the stew, then place over medium low flame and simmer until heated through. Add the beef and simmer. Adjust seasoning with salt, then stir in the lemon juice and serve.

CHAPTER 6

Side Dish Recipes

Tender Roasted Sweet Potatoes with Savory Tahini Sauce

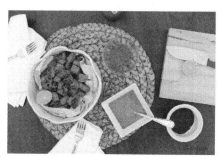

Makes: 8 servings

Ingredients:

❖ 4 large sweet potatoes, peeled and sliced into half-inch thick coins

❖ 6 Tbsp. tamarind syrup

❖ 4 Tbsp. chopped fresh cilantro

❖ Sea salt

❖ Extra virgin olive oil

For the Savory Tahini Sauce:

❖ 1 1/2 cups tahini

❖ 1 1/2 Tbsp. freshly squeezed lemon juice

- ❖ 1 1/2 Tbsp. Greek yogurt
- ❖ 1 1/2 cups water
- ❖ 3 garlic cloves, grated
- ❖ Sea salt

Instructions:

1. First make the tahini sauce by combining all of the ingredients in a bowl and whisking vigorously until creamy. Cover and refrigerate until ready to serve.

2. Set the oven to 450 degrees F. Line a baking sheet with baking paper and set aside.

3. Place the sweet potatoes in a bowl, then drizzle in a bit of olive oil and sprinkle with salt. Spread out on the prepared baking sheet in a single layer, then roast for up to 30 minutes, or until tender and browned.

4. Transfer the roasted sweet potatoes on a serving dish, then spoon the tahini sauce and tamarind syrup on top.

5. Add a drizzle of olive oil, season lightly with salt, garnish with cilantro, then serve right away.

Homemade Whole Wheat Pita Bread

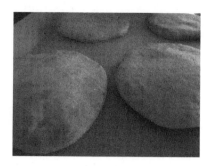

Makes: 12 pieces

Ingredients:

* ❖ 4 cups whole wheat flour (or gluten-free flour)

* ❖ 3 cups unbleached all-purpose flour (or gluten-free alternative)

* ❖ 2 1/4 cups warm water

* ❖ 2 Tbsp. active dry yeast

* ❖ 2 Tbsp. extra virgin olive oil

* ❖ 1 Tbsp. sea salt

Instructions:

1. Combine the yeast and warm water in a very large mixing bowl until thoroughly combined. Stir in the salt.

2. Gradually stir in the two flours into the mixture until you get a dough.

3. Lightly flour a clean, dry surface and place the dough on top. Knead until the dough becomes smooth.

4. Add the olive oil into a large bowl and place the dough on top. Turn the dough several times to coat in the oil. Lightly oil one side of a sheet of plastic wrap, then cover over the bowl. Place a clean kitchen towel over the bowl, then set aside for about 2 hours to rise.

5. Punch down on the risen dough, then divide into 12 pieces. Roll up into balls and arrange on a lightly floured surface. Cover with a clean kitchen towel and allow to rise for about 15 minutes.

6. Set the oven to 475 degrees F. Place a baking sheet on the lowest rack inside.

7. Roll out each ball of dough until each is approximately 6 inches in diameter. Take the baking sheet out of the oven and arrange the unbaked pita on top; do not overcrowd. Bake in batches, if needed.

8. Bake for 12 minutes, then place on a platter. Consume within 3 days.

Crisp Spiced Cauliflower with Feta Cheese

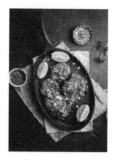

Makes: 4 servings

Ingredients:

- ❖ 3/4 lb cauliflower, chopped

- ❖ 1/2 Tbsp. ground toasted cumin seeds

- ❖ 1 garlic clove, grated

- ❖ 2 Tbsp. crumbled feta cheese

- ❖ 1 1/2 Tbsp. freshly squeezed lemon juice

- ❖ 1 Tbsp. chopped fresh flat leaf parsley

- ❖ Chili flakes

- ❖ Sweet smoked paprika

- ❖ Sea salt

- ❖ Canola oil

Instructions:

1. Place a skillet over high flame and heat just enough canola oil to cover the bottom.

2. Allow the oil to smoke slightly, then add the chopped cauliflower and stir fry for about 2 minutes or until browned and crisp. Season with salt.

3. Reduce to medium flame as you continue to stir fry the cauliflower. Sprinkle in the cumin, lemon juice, grated garlic, and a dash of chili flakes, then stir well to combine.

4. Transfer the cauliflower to a platter, then top with feta, parsley, and a dash of paprika. Serve right away.

Pumpkin Kibbeh

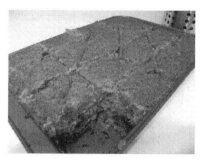

Makes: 4 servings

Ingredients:

- ❖ 1 lb cooked pumpkin chunks

- ❖ 1 cup cooked garbanzo beans (chickpeas)

- ❖ 3/4 cup fine bulgur (or quinoa)

- ❖ 1/2 lb fresh spinach, rinsed

- ❖ 1/2 cup fresh bread crumbs

- ❖ 1 1/2 Tbsp. sumac

- ❖ 1 large onion, chopped

- ❖ 2 Tbsp. extra virgin olive oil

- ❖ 1/2 tsp. ground cinnamon

- ❖ 1/2 tsp. cumin

- ❖ 1 tsp. paprika

- ❖ 1/2 tsp. dried coriander

- ❖ 1/2 tsp. allspice

❖ 1/2 tsp. sea salt

❖ 1/8 tsp. freshly ground white pepper

❖ 2 1/2 Tbsp. toasted pine nuts

Instructions:

1. Place the bulgur in a mesh strainer and rinse thoroughly. Transfer to a bowl, then pour just enough water to cover it by about an inch. Set aside for 5 minutes to fluff up. Drain excess liquid, then set aside.

2. Place a saucepan over medium flame and heat a tablespoon of olive oil. Saute the onion until translucent, then stir in the spinach and cook until wilted. Turn off the heat.

3. Add the garbanzo beans and mix well, then fold in the white pepper, salt, and sumac.

4. Set the oven to 350 degrees F. Lightly coat a baking pan with olive oil and set aside.

5. In a mixing bowl, combined the pumpkin chunks and bulgur, then fold in the bread crumbs, cumin, cinnamon, paprika, allspice, and dried coriander.

6. Pack half of the pumpkin and bulgur mixture into the prepared baking pan, then spread the onion and spinach mixture on top. Add the rest of the pumpkin and bulgur mixture and pack well.

7. Using a sharp knife, score the top of the mixture, then sprinkle the pine nuts over everything and drizzle the rest of the olive oil on top.

8. Bake for 20 to 30 minutes, or until the mixture is golden brown. Serve warm.

Oven Roasted Carrots with Olives and Cumin Yogurt Sauce

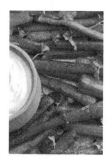

Makes: 8 servings

Ingredients:

- ❖ 30 baby carrots, scrubbed

- ❖ 1/2 cup pitted and halved black olives, oil-cured

- ❖ 1/2 cup Greek yogurt

- ❖ 4 tsp. freshly ground toasted cumin seeds

- ❖ 2 Tbsp. chopped fresh cilantro

- ❖ 6 fresh thyme sprigs

- ❖ 2 Tbsp. freshly squeezed lemon juice

- ❖ Sea salt

- ❖ Freshly ground black pepper

- ❖ Canola oil

- ❖ Extra virgin olive oil

Instructions:

1. First, combine the yogurt with the cumin, cilantro, and lemon juice in a bowl. Cover and refrigerate until ready to be served.

2. Set the oven to 450 degrees F. Line a baking sheet with baking paper and set aside.

3. Combine the carrot and thyme sprigs in a bowl and add just enough canola oil to lightly coat them. Season with salt.

4. Spread the carrot mixture on the prepared baking sheet in a single layer, then roast for up to 30 minutes, or until lightly browned and tender.

5. Carefully remove the baking sheet from the oven and take out the thyme sprigs. Place the carrots on a platter, then spoon the cumin yogurt sauce on top.

6. Sprinkle the olives over the carrot mixture, then drizzle a bit of olive oil over everything and season with salt and pepper. Serve right away.

Bravas Potatoes with Roasted Tomato Sauce

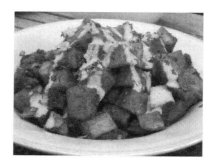

Makes: 6 servings

Ingredients:

- ❖ 3 large Russet potatoes, peeled and cubed

- ❖ 2 medium plum tomatoes

- ❖ 3 garlic cloves, minced

- ❖ 3/4 cup high quality mayonnaise

- ❖ 1 1/2 Tbsp. smoked paprika

- ❖ 1 1/2 Tbsp. sherry vinegar

- ❖ Sea salt

- ❖ Freshly ground black pepper

- ❖ Fresh flat leaf parsley

- ❖ Hot pepper sauce

- ❖ Pure olive oil

Instructions:

1. Set the oven to 425 degrees F.

2. Slice the tomatoes in half and remove the seeds. Place on a baking sheet and roast for 15 minutes, or until tender. Transfer to a cooling rack.

3. Set the oven to 375 degrees F. Put a baking sheet in the middle rack.

4. Pour water into a saucepan until it is about 75 percent full. Place the cubed potatoes inside and add a generous pinch of salt. Place over high flame and boil, uncovered.

5. Once boiling, reduce to medium flame and simmer for up to 10 minutes, or until fork tender. Drain thoroughly and set aside.

6. Place a skillet over medium flame and heat 1 1/2 tablespoons of olive oil. Saute the garlic until fragrant, then stir in the paprika and saute until fragrant. Turn off the heat and let stand until cooled slightly.

7. Place the roasted tomato halves in the food processor and add the sherry vinegar, garlic and paprika in oil, and a few drops of hot pepper sauce. Blend until smooth. Season to taste with salt and pepper.

8. Place a heavy duty skillet over medium flame and pour in enough olive oil until it is about 2 inches deep. Heat until the temperature is at about 300 degrees F. Deep fry the cubed potatoes until golden brown all over. Transfer to a plate lined with paper towels to drain.

9. Transfer the drained potato into a mixing bowl and lightly season to taste with salt and pepper.

10. Take the baking sheet out of the oven and spread the potatoes on it in an even layer. Bake for 10 minutes, or until crisp.

11. Transfer the potatoes to a platter and spoon the roasted tomato sauce on top. Garnish with parsley, then serve right away.

Spring Peas and Beans with Zesty Thyme Yogurt Sauce

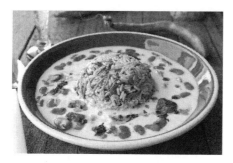

Makes: 4 servings

Ingredients:

- ❖ 3/4 lb fresh shelling beans, shelled

- ❖ 3/4 lb fresh peas (such as English peas, edamame, etc.), shelled

- ❖ 1 lb pole beans, preferably assorted (such as purple wax, Romano, and yellow)

- ❖ 6 young pea shoots

- ❖ 1/2 tsp. ground sumac

- ❖ 1 1/2 Tbsp. extra virgin olive oil

- ❖ Sea salt

For the Zesty Thyme Yogurt Sauce:

- ❖ 1/4 cup Greek yogurt

- ❖ 1 1/2 Tbsp. fresh thyme leaves

- ❖ 1 garlic clove, grated

- ❖ 1/2 lemon, juiced and zested

- ❖ Cayenne

- ❖ Sea salt

Instructions:

1. Combine all the ingredients for the yogurt sauce in a bowl, then season to taste with salt and cayenne. Cover the bowl and refrigerate until ready to serve.

2. Prepare a bowl of ice water and set aside.

3. Boil some salted water in a saucepan, then add the fresh beans and peas. Boil for 2 minutes, or until tender, then remove immediately with a metal mesh strainer and plunge into the ice water to prevent them from being soggy.

4. Blot the peas and beans dry using paper towels, then place in a large bowl and set aside.

5. Refill the bowl of ice water.

6. Boil the salted water in the saucepan again, then add the pole beans and cook for 2 minutes or until almost tender. Remove immediately with a metal mesh strainer and plunge into the ice water to prevent them from being soggy.

7. Blot the pole beans dry using paper towels, then add to the bowl of peas and beans. Toss everything to combine.

8. Drizzle the olive oil over the peas and beans, then season with salt and sumac. Toss well to combine, then add the yogurt sauce on top. Garnish with pea shoots and thyme, then serve right away.

Conclusion

Thank you again for purchasing this book!

I hope this book was able to help you to get started on the Mediterranean diet.

The next step is to stay motivated to live the Mediterranean lifestyle by making it a habit to plan your meals ahead. Find the time to prepare your own dishes and make cooking an enjoyable part of your day. Remember to have fun and let the Mediterranean diet and overall lifestyle inspire you always.

Finally, if you enjoyed this book, please take the time to share your thoughts and post a review on Amazon. I want to reach as many people as I can with this book, and more reviews will help me accomplish that. It'd be greatly appreciated!

Thank you and good luck!

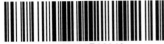

Made in the USA
San Bernardino, CA
25 January 2018